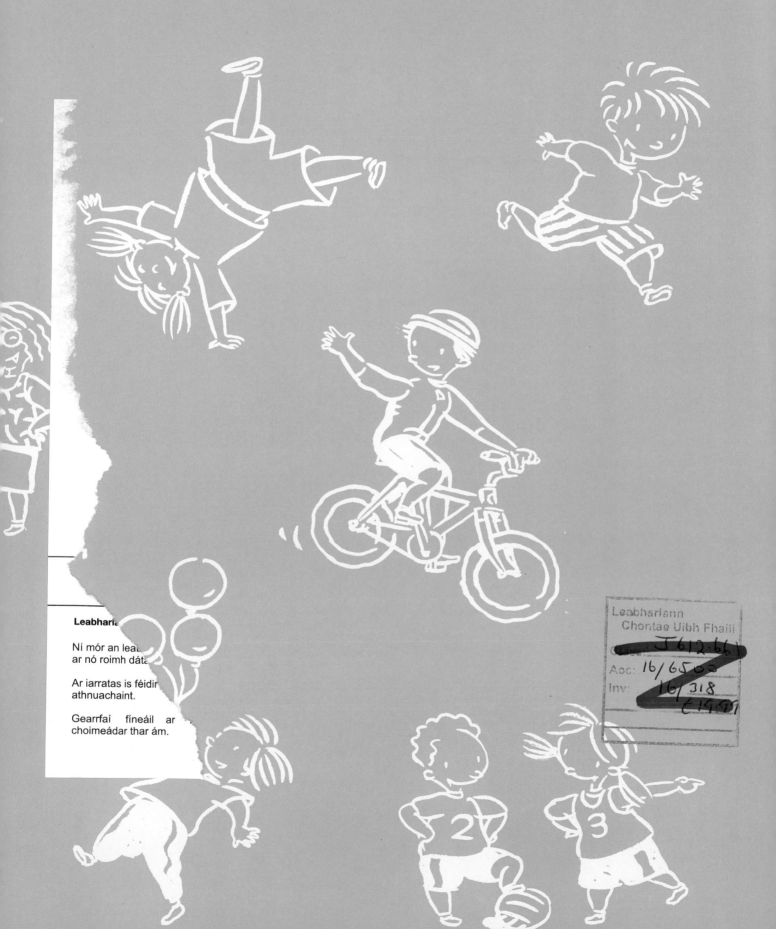

Boys, Girls & Body Science

A First Book about Facts of Life

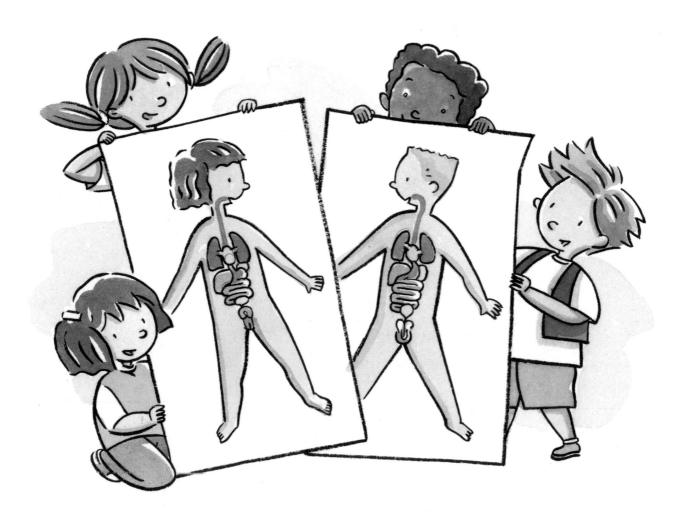

By Meg Hickling

Illustrations by Kim La Fave

Harbour Publishing

The students in Mrs. Miwa's class were really excited. Lots of mums and dads were visiting. Jordan's granddad was there. Maria's foster dad had come too. This day was a special day. They were having a special visitor. Her name was Meg.

"I am a nurse," Meg told them. "I'm here to talk about how our bodies work and how to take good care of them. This is called 'Body Science'."

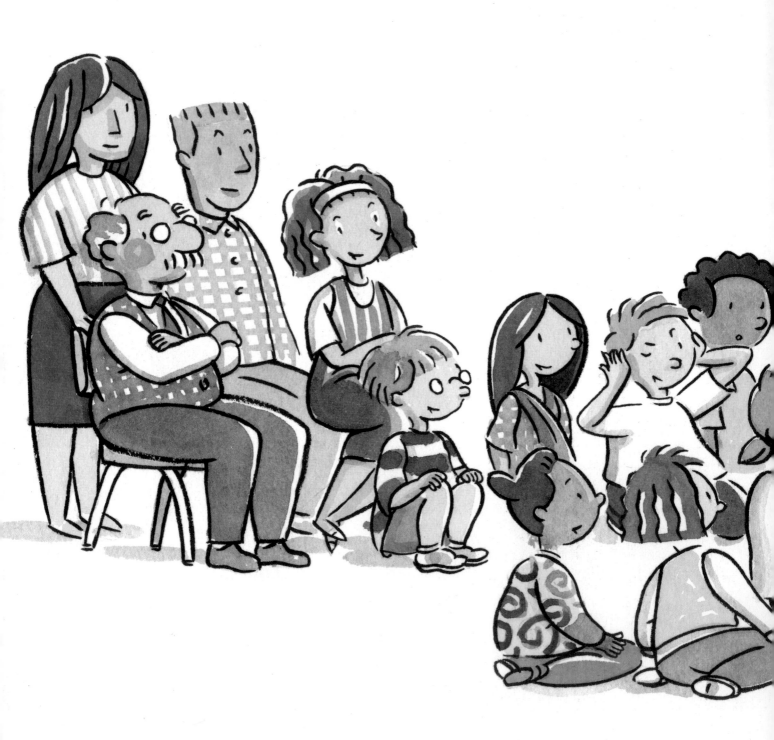

"We've DONE Body Science already," groaned Melanie.

"Yeah, and it was yucky," said Zack.

"Like what happens to food when you swallow it," Satinder said.

"Today we will be talking about a different kind of body science," Meg went on. "Today we will be talking about the parts of our bodies we call our 'private parts'."

"YUCK!" said Zack.

Tim put his hands over his ears.

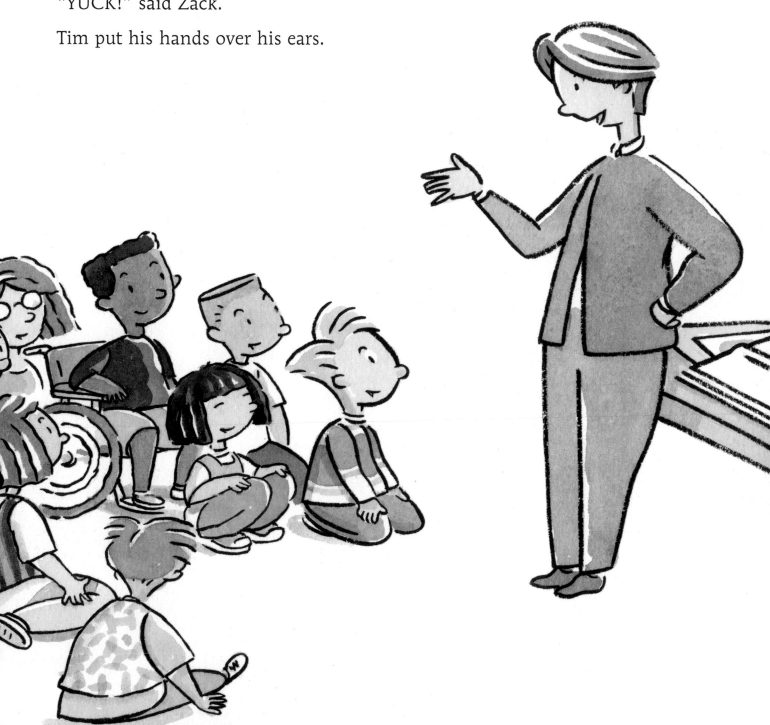

"Talking about private parts sometimes makes us feel embarrassed," Meg said. "That's why I want to teach you how to think like scientists."

She explained that scientists have special scientific words that let us talk about embarrassing things without feeling shy.

Tim took one hand off an ear but left the other one there, just in case.

"And do you know one thing that scientists never do?" asked Meg.

"Tell us, Meg!" said Zack.

"Scientists never say 'Yuck'," said Meg. "Instead, they say 'In-ter-es-ting!'"

"Interesting!" said the children and adults.

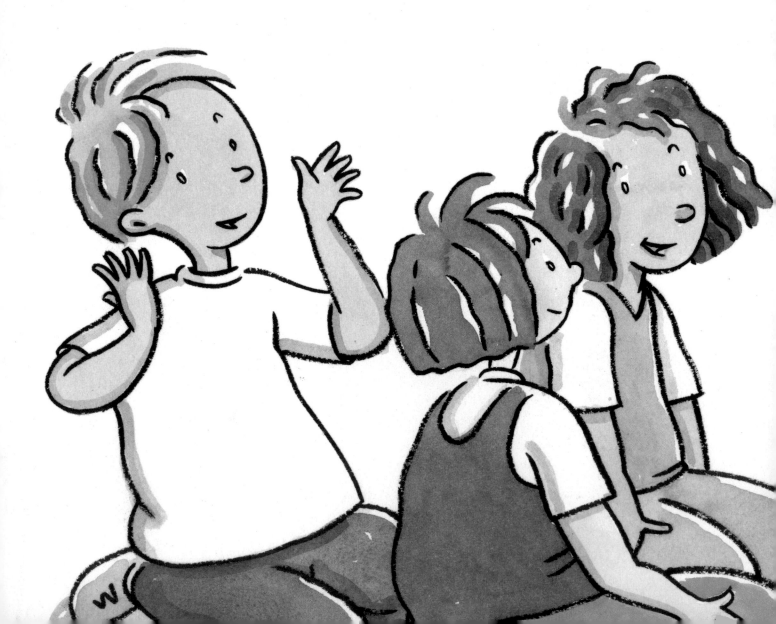

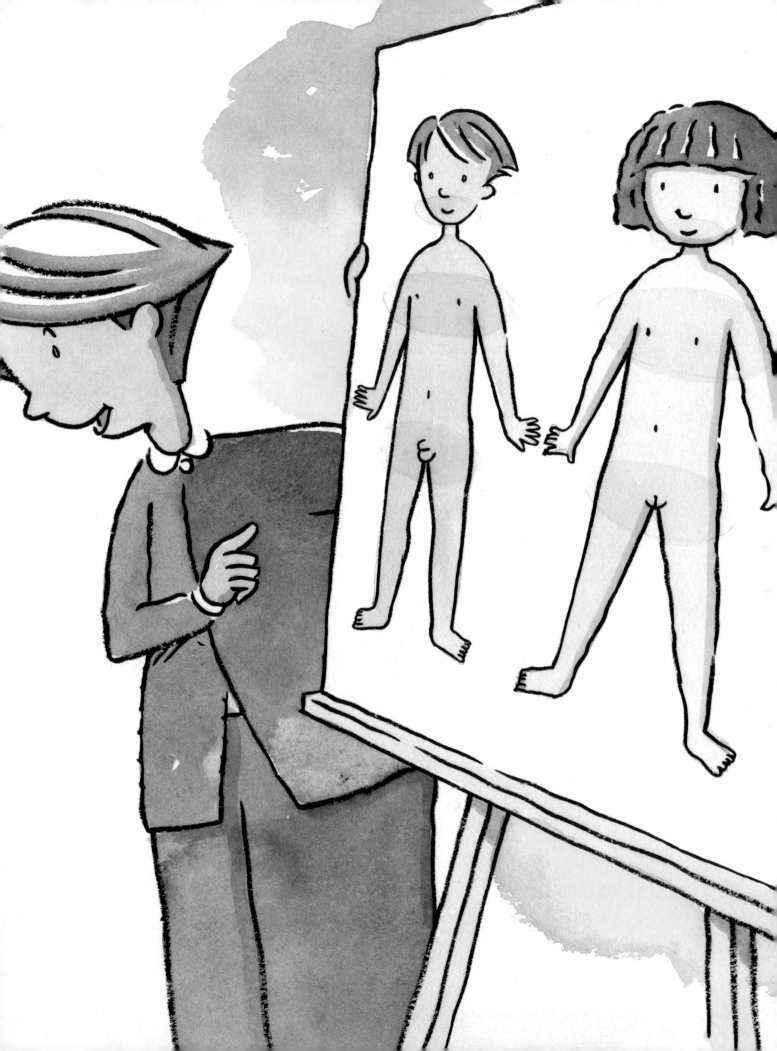

"Excellent," said Meg. "You have made the first step to becoming scientists."

There are three parts of your body that are called private, Meg told them. One part is your mouth. That means that you don't have to have kisses that you don't want.

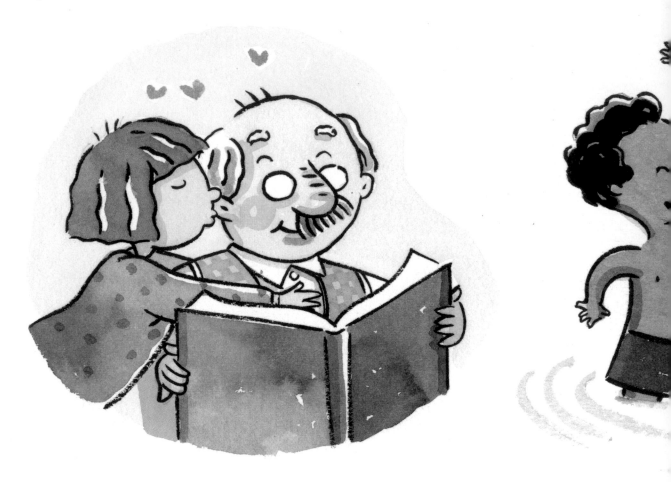

"But I like good-night kisses," said Ming.

"That's wonderful," said Meg. "But if someone you don't want to kiss tries it, you can say 'No.'

"Another part that is private is the breast area and it is private for boys and for girls," Meg said.

"No pinching nipples," shouted Eric.

Mrs. Miwa told them the person who says 'no touching' always rules.

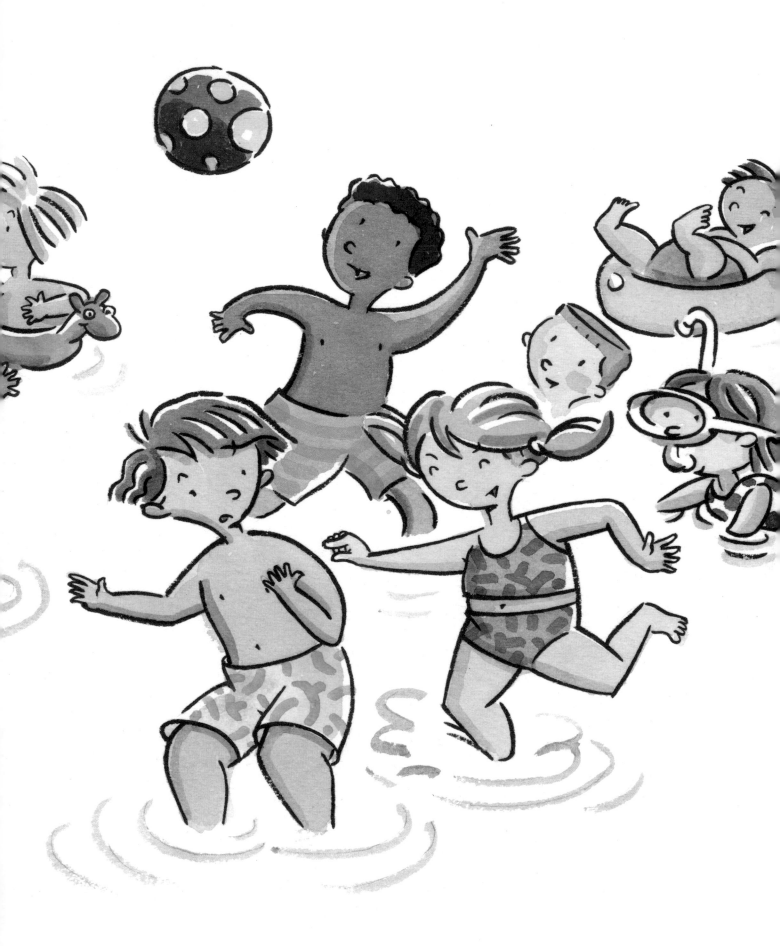

"Now does anyone know where the last parts are that are private?"

Some children nodded and some giggled.

"Between the LEGS!" shouted Eric.

"That's right," said Meg. "Scientists call the area between the legs the genital area." Then she got everyone to say "genital," and told them more about the genital area.

When you are having a bath or shower, you must wash your genital area and look at it to make sure it is healthy. It is not supposed to be private from you. If you have a genital problem, you shouldn't be afraid to tell your parents, the nurse or doctor.

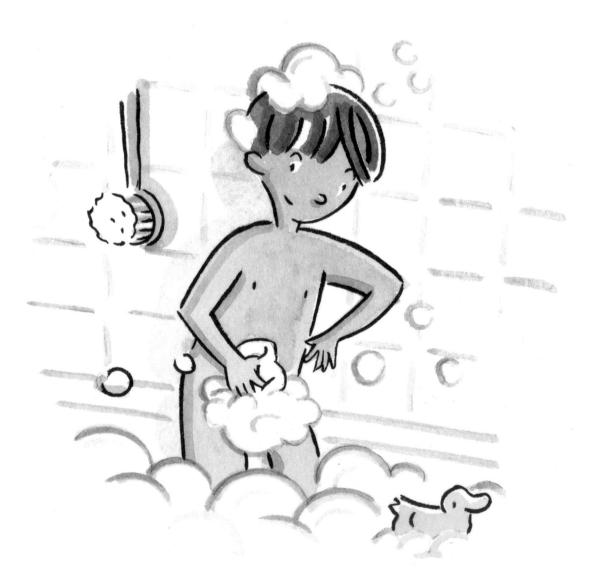

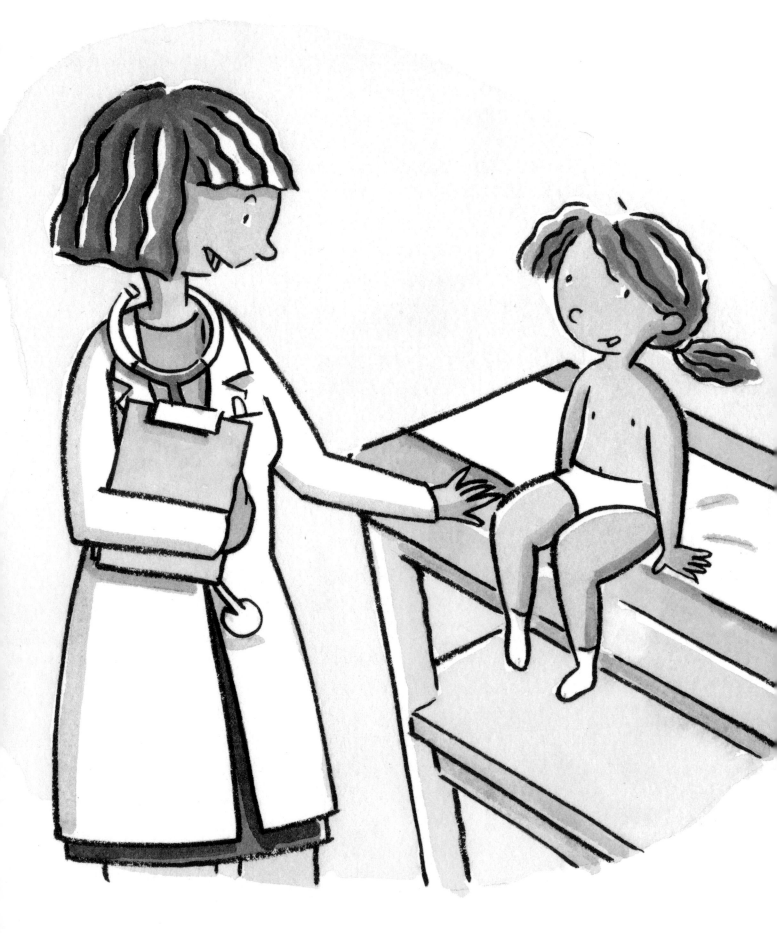

"Now," said Meg, "let's learn some more body science."

The class had already learned that the body makes two kinds of waste, the solid kind and the watery kind. The solid kind is called stool and it leaves the body from an opening behind the genital area called the anus. Watery waste is called urine and collects in a stretchy bag called the bladder.

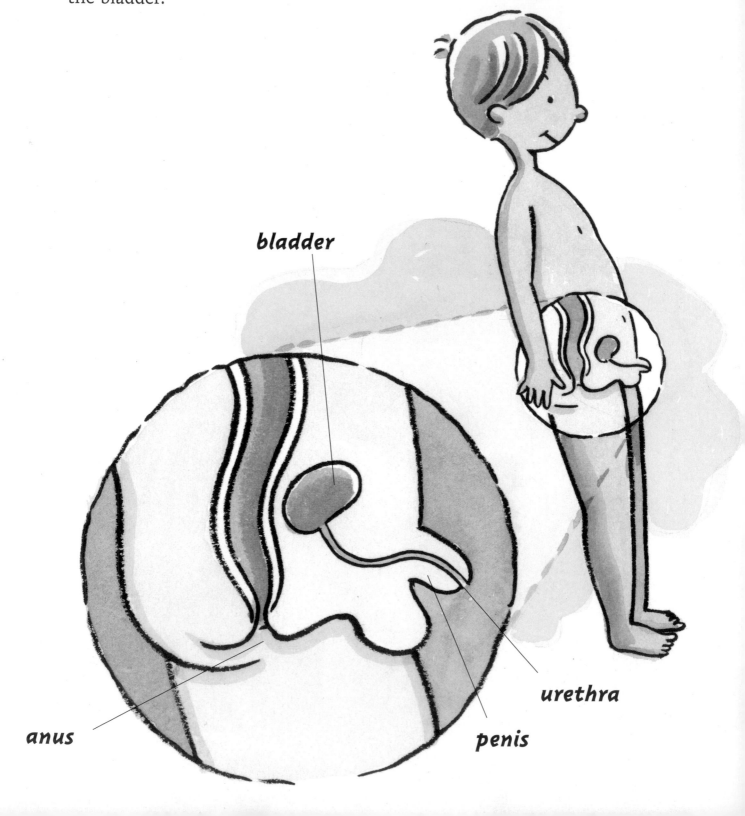

bladder

anus

penis

urethra

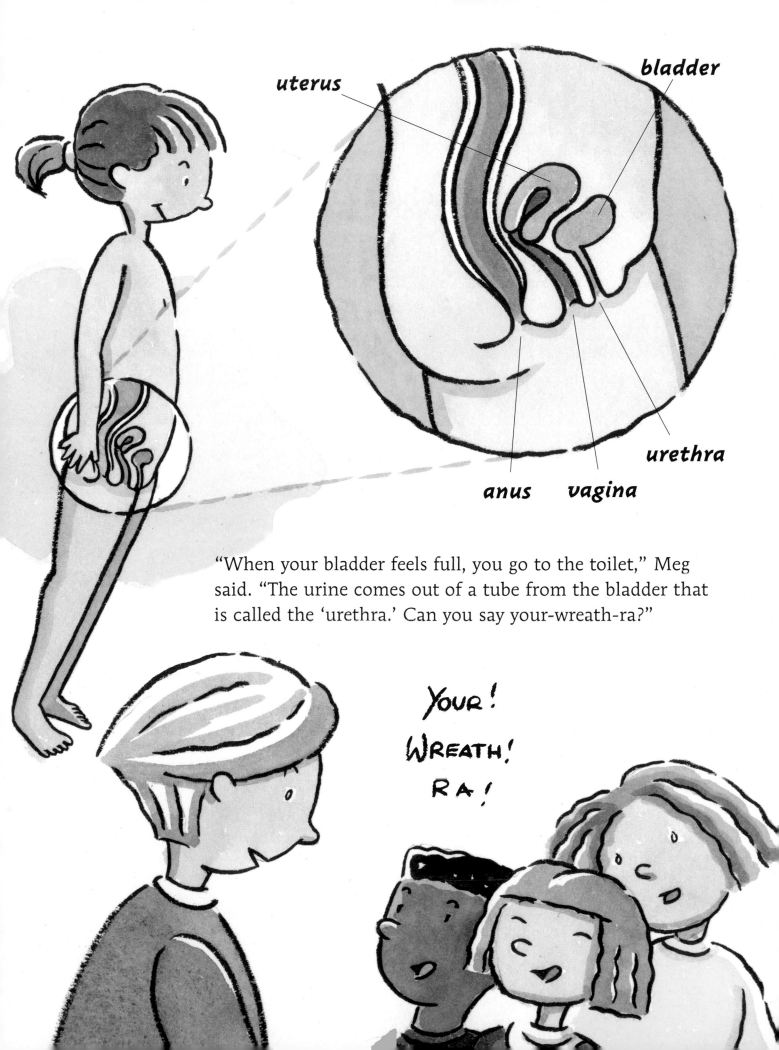

uterus

bladder

anus   vagina   urethra

"When your bladder feels full, you go to the toilet," Meg said. "The urine comes out of a tube from the bladder that is called the 'urethra.' Can you say your-wreath-ra?"

YOUR!
WREATH!
RA!

"You are such good scientists," said Meg. "Now, can you tell me where the urethra comes out?"

"My granddad calls it your pee-pee," Jordan said.

Some of the other children laughed.

"Well, in the olden days," Meg explained, "children didn't have Body Science lessons and they didn't learn the scientific names. Does anyone know the scientific name for a boy's pee-pee?"

"Penis!" said Yuki.

"That is correct," said Meg. "Let's learn more. Behind the penis, between the boy's legs, is a little bag of wrinkly skin called a scrotum. Can anybody tell me what's inside the scrotum?"

"BALLS!" yelled Eric.

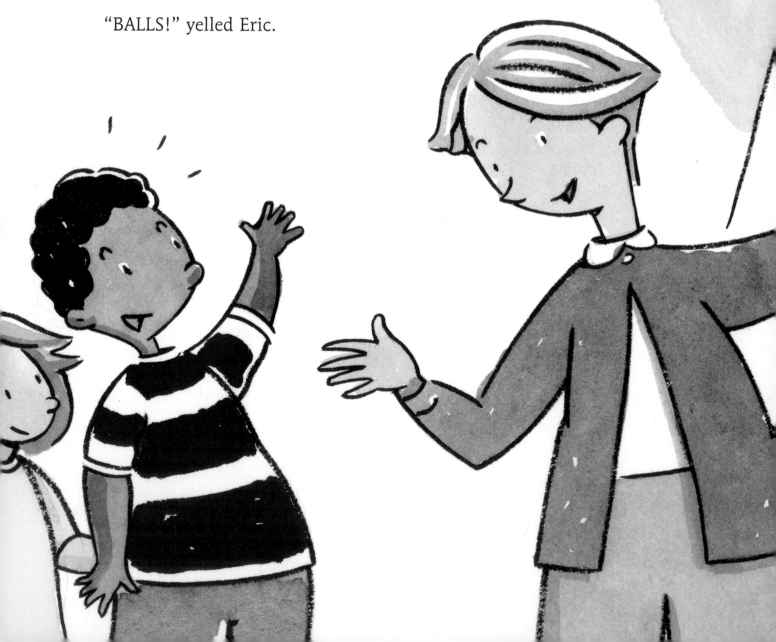

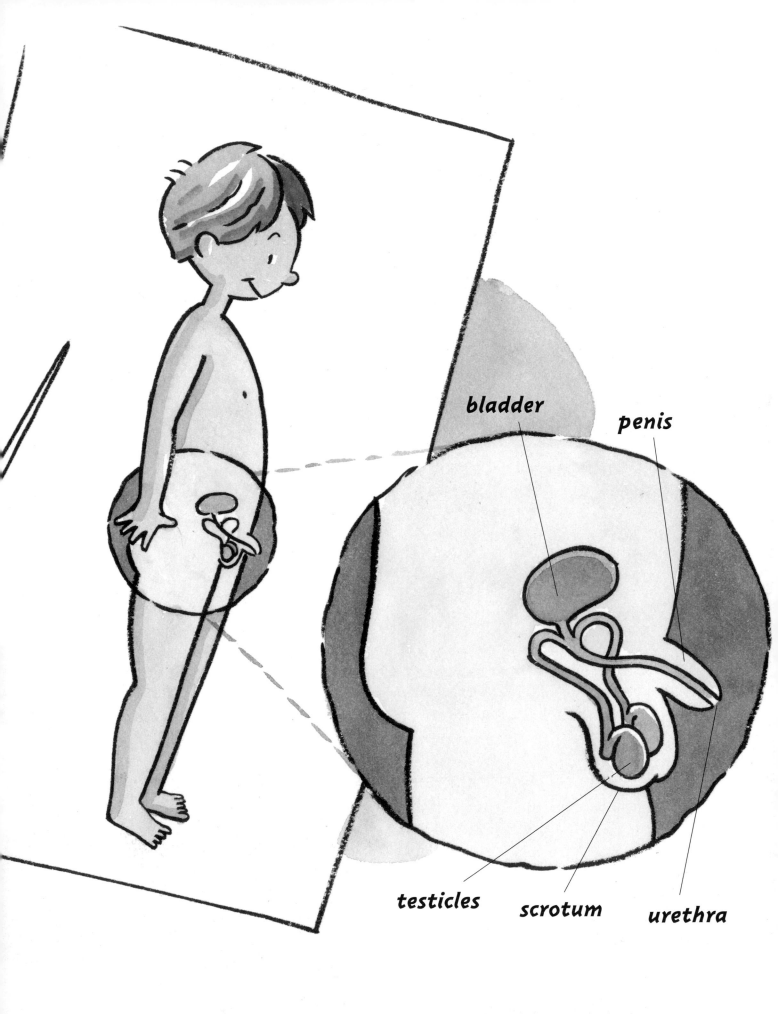

bladder

penis

testicles

scrotum

urethra

"Right," said Meg. "But if you were a scientist, you would call them testicles. They make the boys' growing hormone. It is a little bit like growing-juice, so you have to take good care of your testicles."

"Yes, you have to wear a plastic cup in hockey to protect your testicles," said Zack.

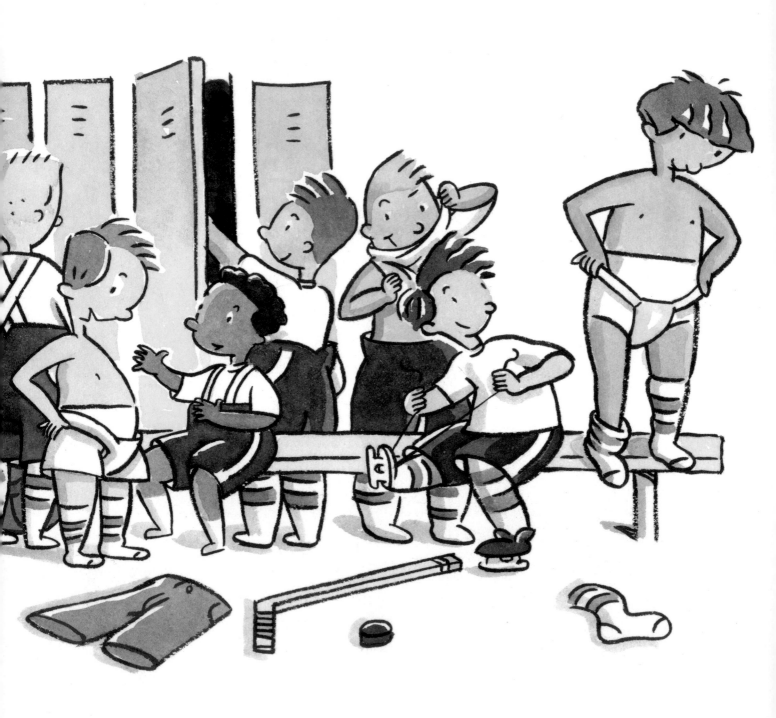

"Very good," said Meg, "and no wedgies! When someone yanks up on a boy's pants, it can damage his genitals. Be sure to tell the nurse, or doctor, or your parents right away if your testicles ever hurt."

"Let's learn more about girls' body science now," said Kim.

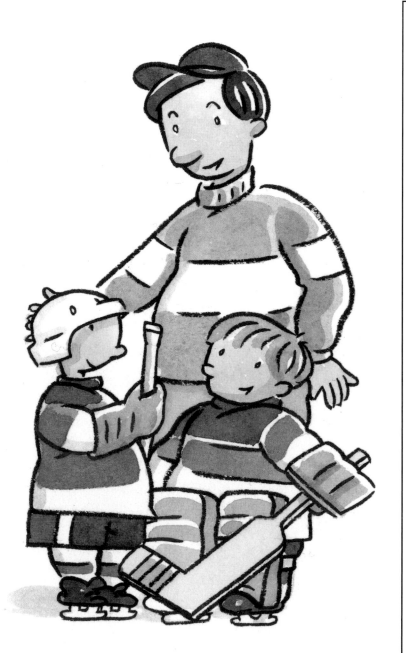

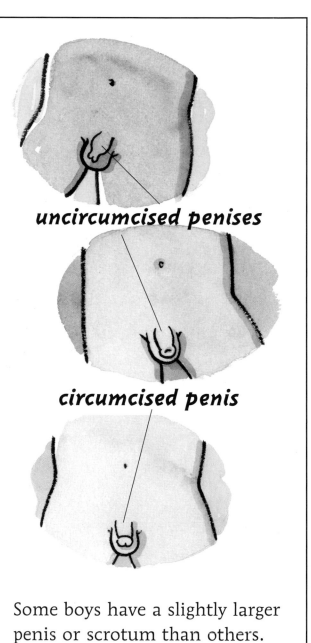

uncircumcised penises

circumcised penis

Some boys have a slightly larger penis or scrotum than others. They appear in many different sizes.

"All right," said Meg. "Girls' genital area is covered by folds of skin called the vulva. Between the folds at the front of the vulva there is the clitoris, about as big as the end of your little finger. It doesn't have an opening, and it feels tickly if you touch it when you are bathing. Let's see if you can tell me something. You know that boys have two openings between their legs, the urethra and the anus. How many openings do girls have?"

"One?" guessed Zack.

"Three!" shouted Jenny and Melanie and Yuki.

"Why do girls need three?" asked Zack.

"I know, I know," said Eric. "Girls have an extra one for the baby to come out."

"You are so right, Eric," said Meg. "It's between the urethra and anus and it's called the vagina. Most of the time it is closed but when the baby is being born it stretches open."

"Do girls have balls?" asked Zack.

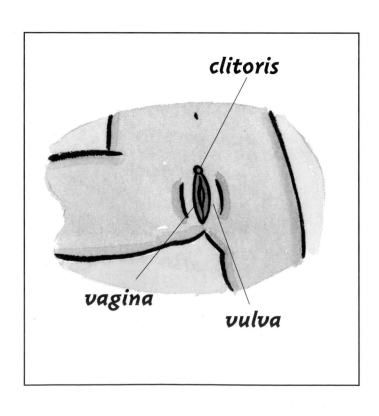

clitoris

vagina

vulva

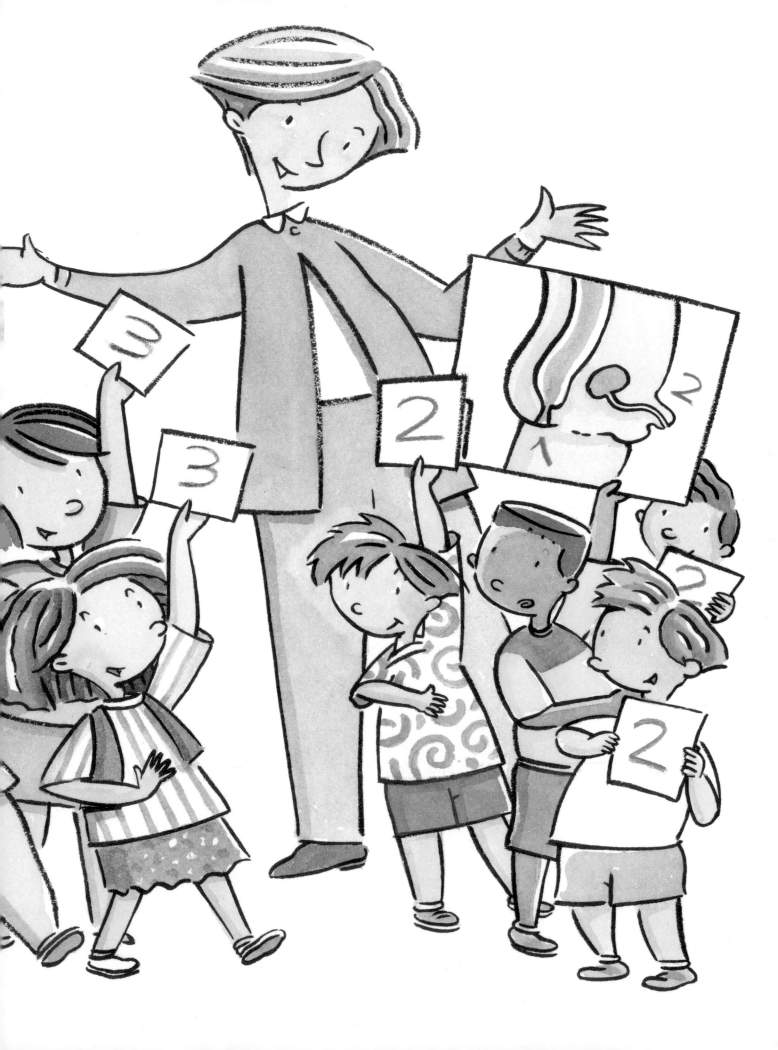

Some children giggled and said "no-o-o," but Meg said, "Well, girls have two ovaries inside their abdomen and they are sort of like balls. Now, who can think like a scientist and tell us what is inside the girls' ovaries?"

"I know," said Satinder, "the eggs to make babies."

"Let me shake your hand," said Meg. "Making babies is just what we are going to talk about next."

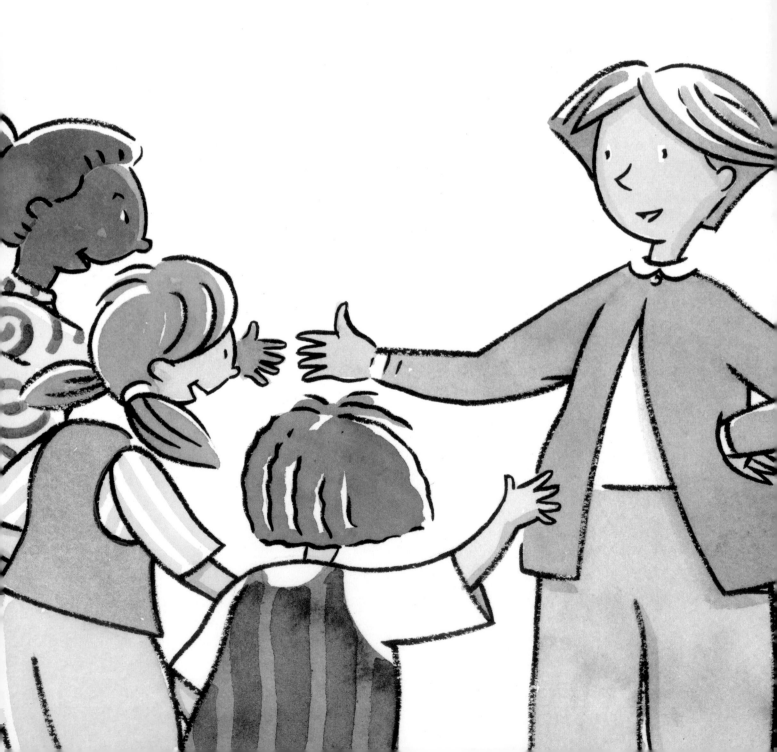

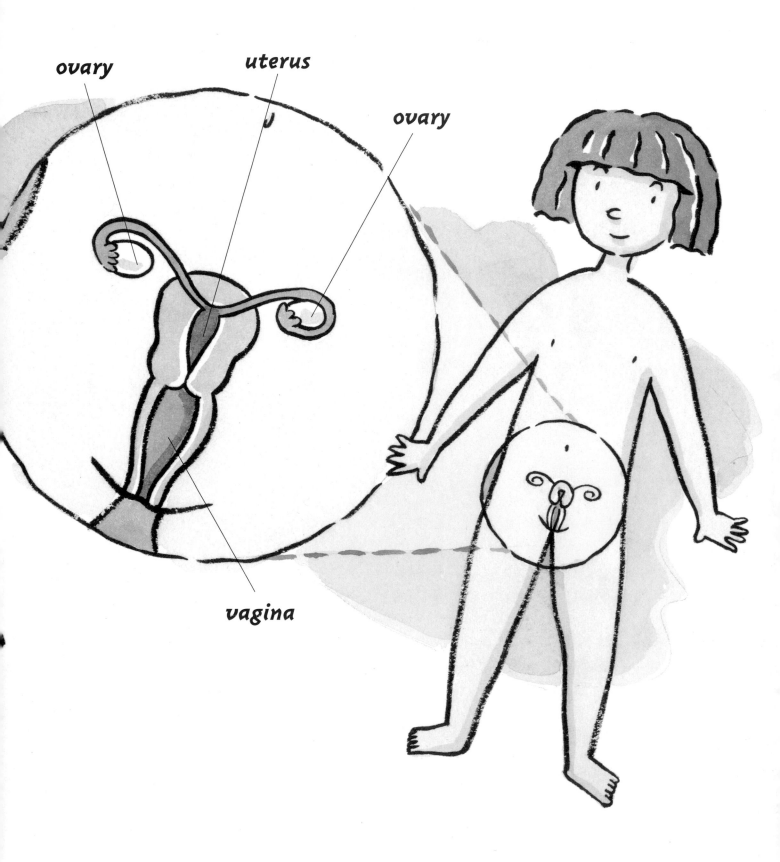

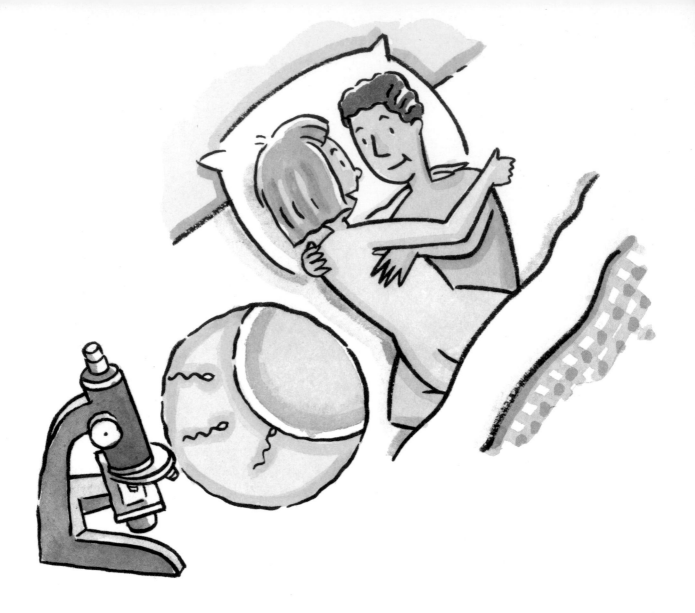

When two adults want to make a baby, Meg told the class, they must wait until the mother's ovary sends out an egg cell. It is only the size of a grain of sand and is called an ovum, but it will not start growing into a baby on its own. First it must be joined by a sperm cell made in the father's testicles. These sperm cells are so small that you need a micro-scope to see them, and the father must use his penis to put them in the mother's vagina. The interesting science is that the father can only do this when his penis gets erect, meaning it grows longer and becomes stiff.

"Interesting," said all the children.

"That's called 'having sex'," said Melanie.

"You are all good body scientists," said Meg. "Boys' penises sometimes have erections just for practice, and that is healthy. But only grown-ups should have sex."

"I am never doing that even when I am grown up," said Satinder. "My mum says you don't have to have sex if you don't want to."

"That's true," said Meg, "and some families say that you should be married first, before you have sex. You need to know the rules for your family."

"My family says no feet on the couch," said Zack.

"My mum said having sex can be really nice when you are grown up," said Jenny.

Ben said, "If you want, you could be a foster parent or you could adopt a baby too."

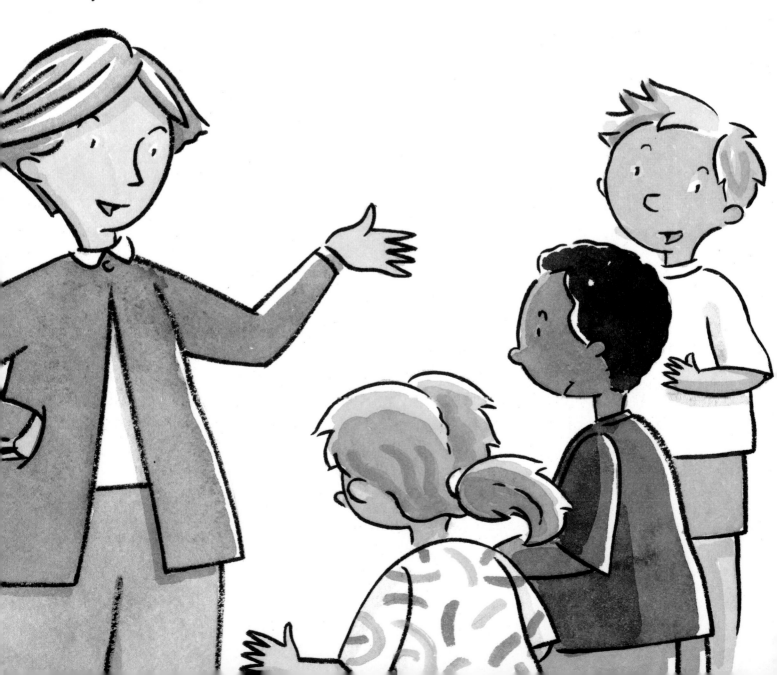

"Now here is a huge science question," said Meg. "Where does the baby grow before it comes out of the vagina?"

"In the stomach," several children said.

"No," said Jenny, "it can't be mixed up with the food."

"So, where does the baby grow, Meg?" asked Zack.

"It grows in a special bag called the uterus or womb," Meg told them. "The uterus is made of powerful muscles and it is just behind the bladder. The lower end of the uterus is connected to the vagina."

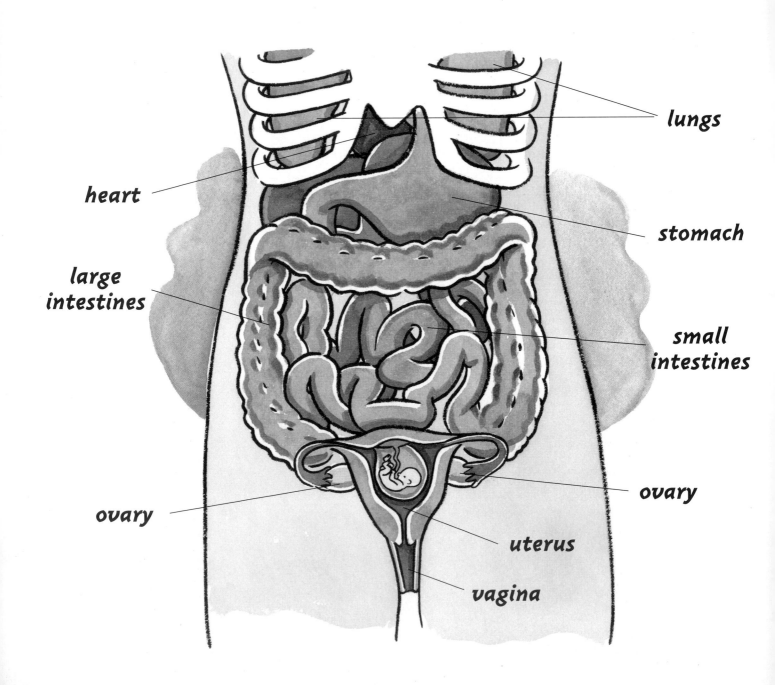

lungs

heart

stomach

large intestines

small intestines

ovary

ovary

uterus

vagina

Meg opened a pop-up book and there was a uterus and a baby about newborn size.

"But, it is upside down," said Ming.

"This is actually right side up for a baby," said Meg.

"Standing on its head!" laughed Ben.

"You're right," said Meg. "And there is a reason in science for this. You see, the baby is also in a water bag, which is inside the uterus."

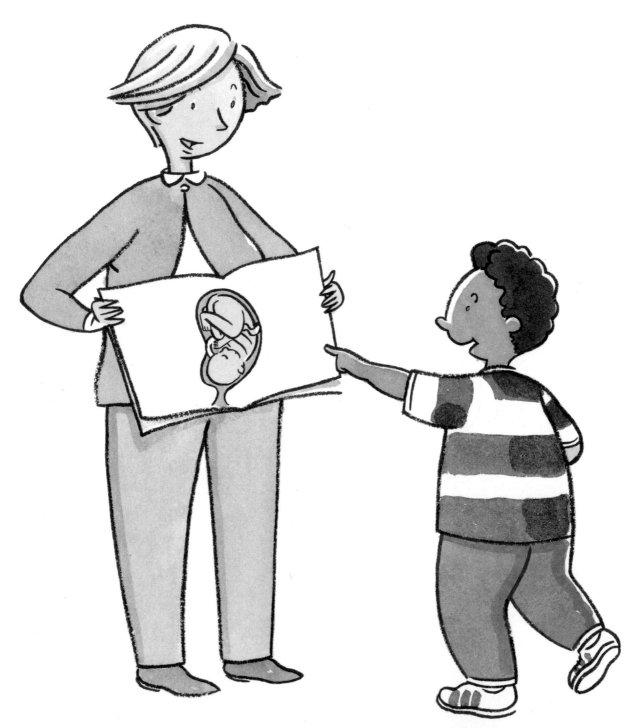

She pointed back at the picture in the pop-up book. The bag looked a bit like a see-through plastic bag. She explained that the water protects the baby in case the mother gets bumped. The baby is upside down because the head is the heaviest part in the water bag.

"But how does the baby breathe?" asked Eric.

"Good question," said Meg. "The baby can't breathe or eat under water but it does get everything it needs from its mother's blood. Mother and baby are joined by a tube called the umbilical cord or umbilicus. One end of this cord is attached to the mother's uterus. Do you know where the other end goes into the baby?"

"At the belly button," said Jordan.

"Exactly right," said Meg. "Now, let's pretend that it is time for the baby to be born."

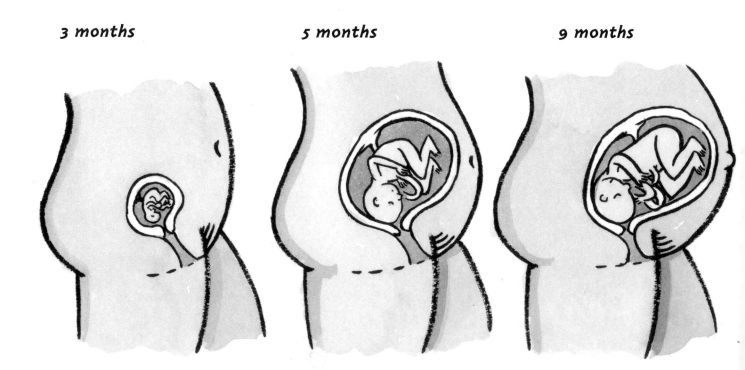

3 months   *5 months*   *9 months*

The mighty muscle of the uterus begins to squeeze, then it relaxes, she told them. A few minutes later it squeezes again and relaxes. It keeps on squeezing and relaxing for many hours. The squeezes or contractions probably feel like giant hugs for the baby and it's these hugs that teach the baby how to breathe.

The children all hugged themselves and said, "Ahh!"

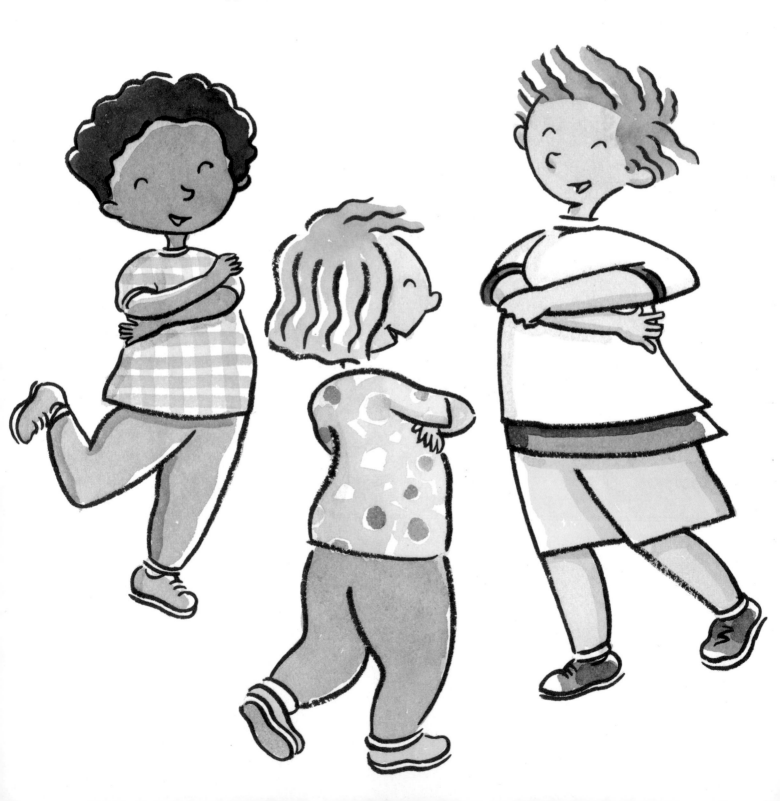

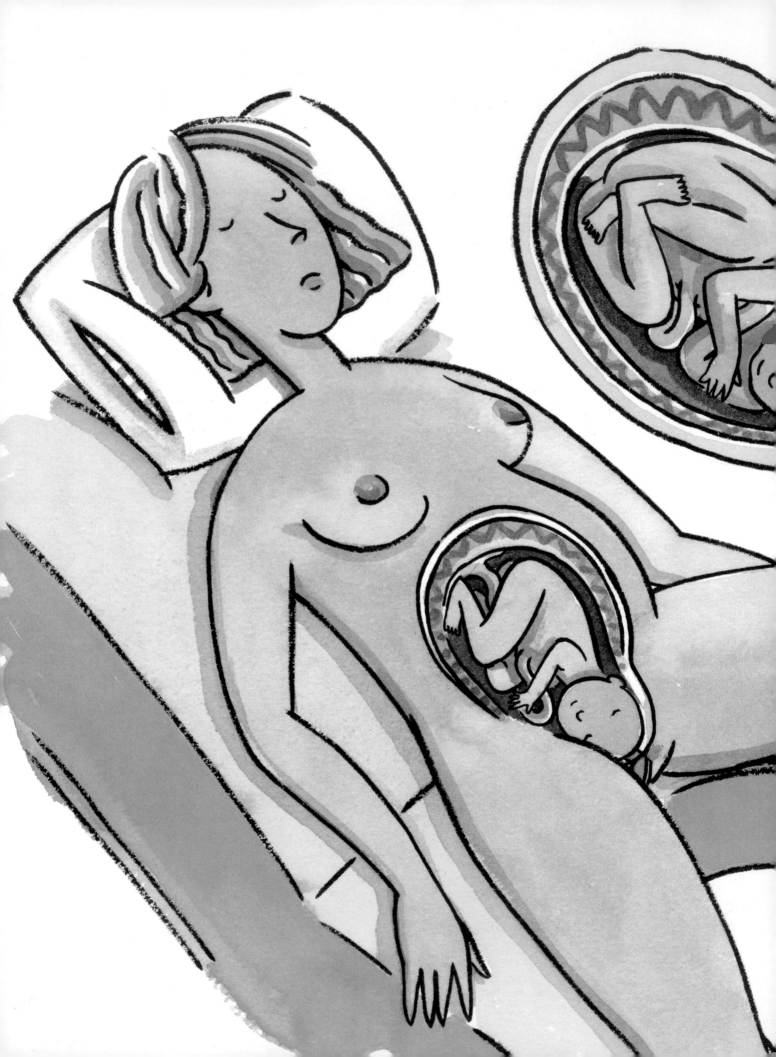

"But what would happen if you kept squeezing on a balloon?" asked Meg.

"It would pop," said Nicholas.

"That is exactly what happens," said Meg. "After a few hours, the water bag breaks and the water comes pouring out of the mum's vagina and makes it all wet and slippery, just like a water slide. So, the first water slide that you ever had was the day you were born when you came slip-sliding down your mum's vagina."

All the children loved the water slide story and made swooshy noises as they waved their arms around.

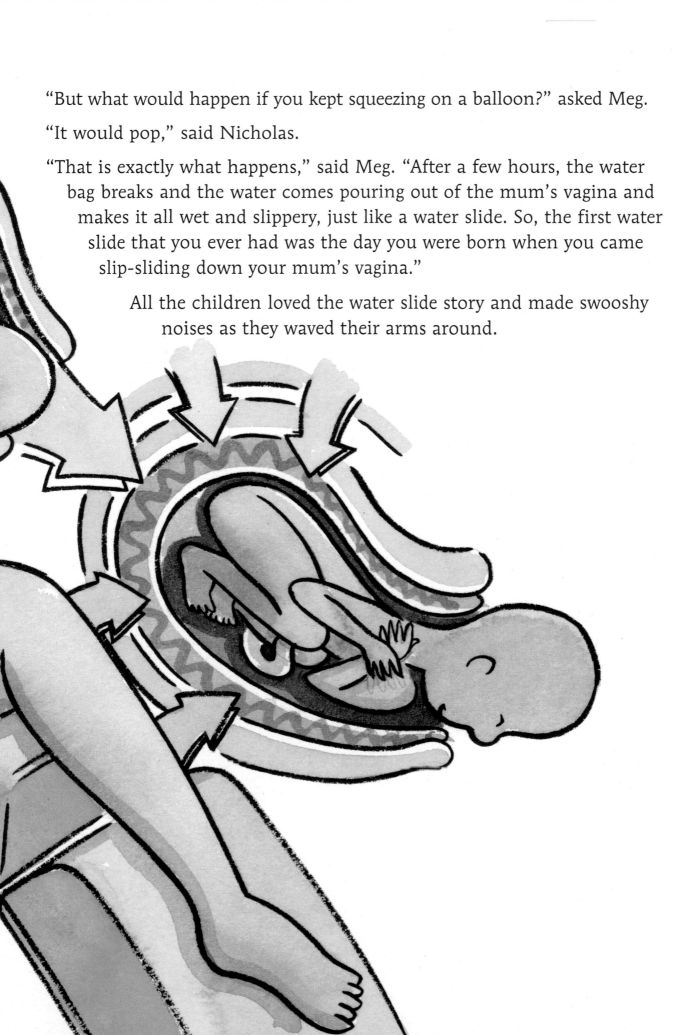

"Some babies and their mums need extra help," explained Meg. "So, the doctor does an operation to cut open the mother's uterus. This operation is called a Caesarean or C-section. Some of you were probably born like that."

"My mum had an operation to get me out," said Melanie.

"When the babies come out," Meg went on, "they begin to breathe and then the umbilical cord can be cut. It doesn't hurt. It's like cutting hair. Later, the place where the cord joined the baby closes itself in a kind of knot. This is how we all got our belly buttons. Some of us have an innie knot and some have an outie."

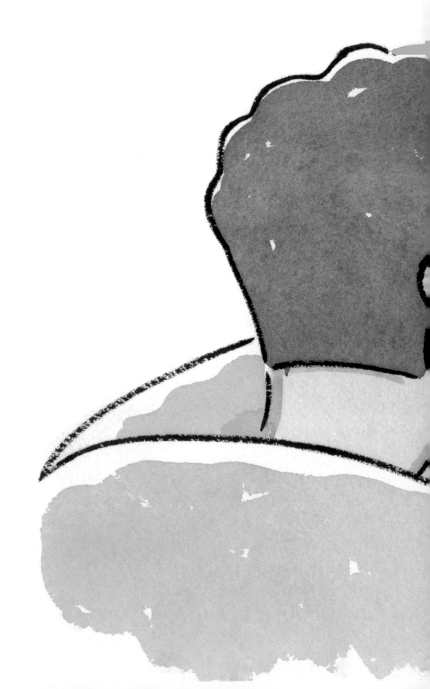

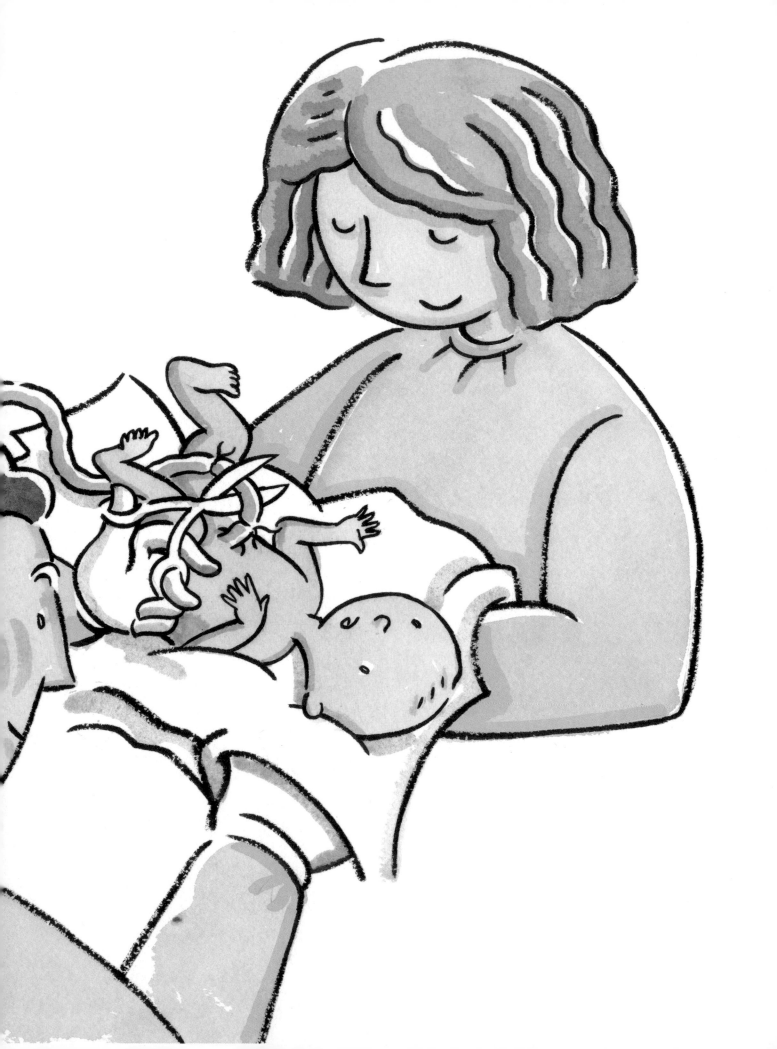

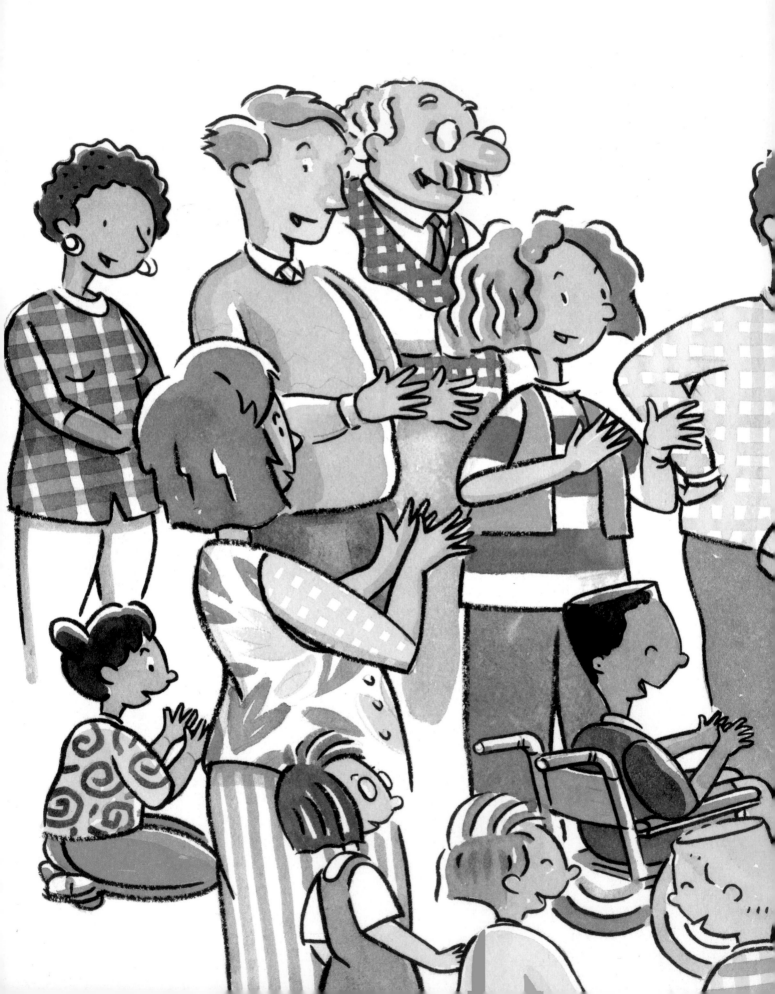

"I have an innie," said Satinder.

"I have an outie," said Eric.

"I have an outie too," said Jenny, "but can we have our snack now?"

"You can," said Mrs. Miwa, "but first, let's thank Meg for coming to Craig Bay School today."

"Thank you, Meg!" everyone said.

"Interesting!" said Tim at the top of his voice.

And the grown-ups all clapped.

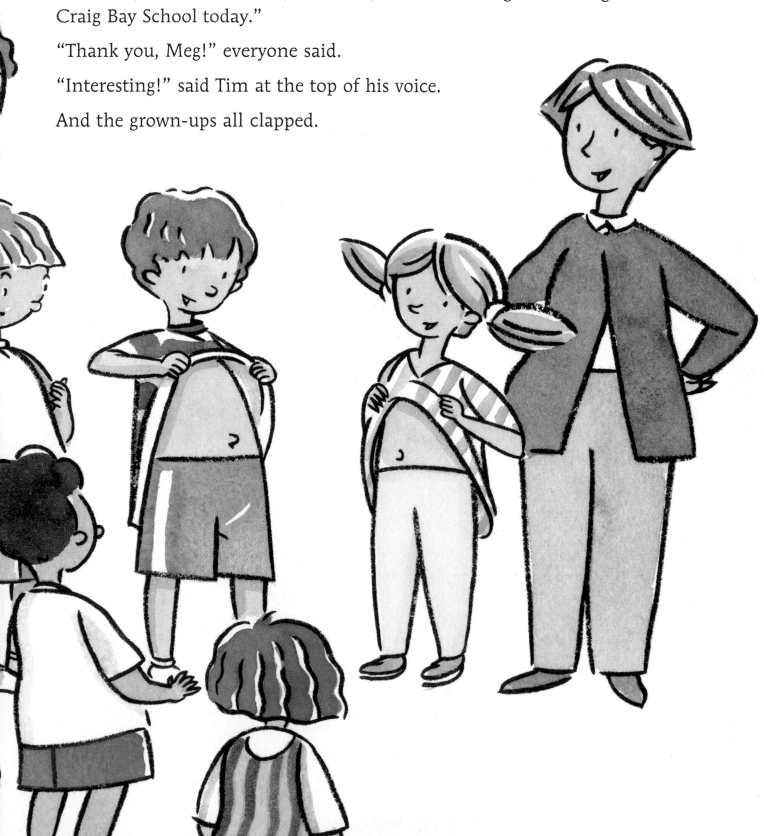

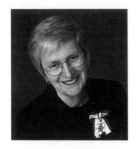

Meg Hickling M.C., O.B.C., L.L.D. (Hon.), R.N. is a registered nurse and best-selling author whose expertise in sexual health education has earned her many honours including an Honorary Doctorate of Laws from the University of British Columbia, the Order of Canada and the Order of British Columbia. She is the author of two books for parents, *Speaking of Sex* and *More Speaking of Sex*. She lives in Vancouver, BC with her husband Tony and has three adult children and two grandchildren.

Kim La Fave is an internationally published illustrator whose books have earned many awards, including the Ruth Schwartz Children's Book Award, the Amelia Frances Howard Gibbon Award and the Governor General's Award. He has two sons and lives in Roberts Creek, BC with his wife, Carol.

Text copyright © 2002 Meg Hickling
Illustrations copyright © 2002 Kim La Fave

10   11   12   13   14   20   19   18   17   16

Published by
HARBOUR PUBLISHING CO. LTD.
P.O. Box 219
Madeira Park, BC Canada
V0N 2H0
www.harbourpublishing.com

Cover and page design by Roger Handling

Printed in China through Colorcraft Ltd, Hong Kong

Harbour Publishing acknowledges financial support from the Government of Canada through the Book Publishing Industry Development Program and the Canada Council for the Arts, and from the Province of British Columbia through the BC Arts Council and the Book Publishing Tax credit.

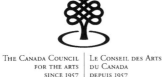

THE CANADA COUNCIL | LE CONSEIL DES ARTS
FOR THE ARTS | DU CANADA
SINCE 1957 | DEPUIS 1957

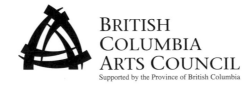

BRITISH COLUMBIA ARTS COUNCIL
Supported by the Province of British Columbia

National Library of Canada Cataloguing in Publication

Hickling, Meg, 1941–
    Boys, girls and body science

    ISBN 1-55017-236-0
    ISBN 978-1-55017-236-2

    1. Sex instruction for children. I. La Fave, Kim. II. Title.
HQ53.H52 2000   j613.9'5   C00-910762-2